DESIGNED
FOR
MOVEMENT

How to Effectively Move
Freely and Live Well

By

ROSEMARY MENDOZA

COPYRIGHT

DISCLAIMER

This book is only intended to provide knowledge that is relevant to daily life. Every effort has been made to provide accurate, current, trustworthy and comprehensive information. Consult your doctor for guidance and counselling.

CONTENTS

Introduction

Chapter 1: Modification Techniques To Broaden The Range of Motion And Prevent Harm

Chapter 2: Integrating More Activity To Your Daily Life Naturally

Chapter 3: Managing Sedentary Behaviors

Chapter 4: Fussy Eaters': No-Fuss Nutrition Guide

Chapter 5: Basic Breathing Techniques For Reducing Tension And Pain

Introduction

Wouldn't fitness, mobility, and longevity be possible if exercise wasn't a barrier? What if we could simply give up the notion of exercising and still feel great, get up and chase the kids, enjoy long, arduous hikes, and play some serious pickup soccer? "Designed for Movement" is a book that aims to persuade us all that exercise is not the solution. There is something a helluva lot more basic and straightforward: Move and continue moving once you stand up.

The entire focus of this book is on helping you remain active well into old age. You'll fare even better if you incorporate regular exercise into the mix. The main point we want to make is that you must move now or continue to move if you want to be able to continue moving as you age. Numerous individuals have staked their reputations on the notion that we should move more throughout the day, in small increments, to achieve our healthiest lifestyles. Sincere introspection, some stretching, and astute body check-ins are the only real ways to enjoy a full physical life. Also necessary is for everyone to celebrate sleeping and walking rather than sitting at desks and working. That is what it is, then.

Exercise is the foundation of fitness, as we've heard over and over again — 150 minutes per week, checked. However, the exercise advice falls apart and the movement ceases for anyone who experiences pain, has difficulty running, is unable to make progress, feels daily dread of working out, or is simply stuck in a rut. We have our priorities backward, which is the problem. Movement, not exercise, should be your compass if you're at sea and feeling thirsty enough to consider drinking salt water. The hidden treasure on the island is more like exercise.

However, how exactly does this appear in more detail? The book "Designed for Movement" is more than just a call to action to get moving; it's also a densely packed, simple-to-follow manual that's full of wise and pragmatist advice. It includes practical sidebars and wonderful, relatable personal anecdotes, as well as everything you'd expect from a good fitness book. We purchase fitness books for a reason, after all. As a result of the fact that we are seeking inspiration, motivation, and a cause to change. This book offers fundamental physical change, and it does so for all the right reasons, for once.

Chapter 1

Modification Techniques to Broaden the Range of Motion and Prevent Harm

How your body moves can be used to describe the Range of Motion (ROM). Each person's version varies and includes both joint and muscular movement. Typically, ROM is evaluated during a physical therapy evaluation or treatment. The body part and individual variations determine normal values. ROM exercises are meant to prevent the onset of contractures, adaptive muscle shortening, and the shortening of the capsule, ligaments, and tendons.

Active and passive ranges of motion can be distinguished from each other.

- When a person moves their body actively, they do so without the aid of an external force. An example of this would be turning to look over your shoulder while doing a quick head check in the car.

- When an external force propels you through a movement, you are said to be in a passive range of motion, which typically denotes a person's full range of motion.

How Is Motion Range Assessed?

To measure a range of motion, some movements are used:

1. Flexion: forward bending motions like chin-to-chest bringing.
2. Extension: bending backward in a way that involves raising your chin high in the air, for example.
3. Rotation: is a turning or twisting motion, like when you check behind you or check inside the car.
4. Lateral Flexion: bringing your ear down to your shoulder is an example.
5. Abduction: is the action of deviating from the midline, as in detaching an arm from the body.

6. Adduction: is the process of bringing an object toward the midline, such as an arm, and body.

Two techniques are used to gauge the range of motion:
1. calculating the percentage difference between benchmarks, which serve as a guide for typical daily movement, and using that number to represent movement loss.
2. utilizing a goniometer that provides a direct angle of movement (best for extremities, such as wrists, knees, etc.)

What Range of Motion Is Deemed To Be "Good"?

Each person's definition of a "good" range of motion will be unique, so we must take into account the joint we are testing for as well as their age, gender, and other factors.

Different joints, like the ankle, have a smaller range of motion and less mobility than joints like the shoulder. As a result, when comparing sides during the range of motion testing, we take into account things like:

Age: In general, the more we age, the more our range of motion decreases and the less movement we typically have.

Gender: The range of motion in females is generally greater than in males. Hormone levels are thought to be the determining factor, and flexibility is becoming increasingly affected by collagen synthesis.

Job: When evaluating a person's range of motion, their job has a significant impact on it and should be taken into account.

Although a person's range of motion can be affected by a variety of factors, many things can be done to increase the range of motion.

How Significant Is A Range Of Motion?

For movement and mobility throughout the entire body, the range of motion is to blame. When we observe a reduction or loss in range of motion, we frequently discover that it can cause pain or irritability, limiting a person's capacity to carry out daily tasks, and resulting in more dysfunction and pain.

Flexibility results in a wide range of motion. A person's ability to perform daily tasks and maintain fitness depend on their flexibility. An exercise program that increases flexibility can enhance range of motion, lessen stiffness and injury, enhance muscular performance, and even elevate your mood.

Why Does A Range of Motion Get Less Or Become Limited?
Many factors can reduce your range of motion, including aging, injury (such as edema, sprains, strains, dislocations, breaks, etc.), immobility, insufficient warm-up and/or cool-down surrounding physical activity, as well as bad postural habits or arthritis/degeneration.

How Can You Increase The Range of Motion In Your Body?
1. Go to a chiropractor

Through the use of manual or low-force adjustments, chiropractors can alleviate tension and restrictions in your joints (most frequently spinal joints). By doing so, you can relieve the tension and stress that has accumulated in your muscles as well as assist the joints move as they should.

How long and the best course of treatment for you will depend on your symptoms when you first arrive, the findings from careful testing, and your ultimate objective.

2. Before exercising, warm up

Before finishing your physical activity, you should do a light and gradual warm-up. To reduce the risk of damage, this helps to gradually boost blood flow while warming up your muscles.

To warm up the muscles targeted for the activity to come, dynamic stretching is often used. A few examples are arm circles, shoulder rolls, arm swings, and leg swings. These facilitate muscle acclimatization and improve performance during exercise.

3. Exercising

You can loosen up your muscles and improve your range of motion by stretching restricted or tight muscles. Which muscles you might need to stretch will depend on the area of the problem. You can develop tailored stretches for your body, your goals, and yourself by seeking the advice of a healthcare professional.

After an activity, while your muscles are already warm, you should perform static stretching as part of your cool-down. A 30-second break should be taken between each stretch.

Static stretching comprises the following examples:

- A hamstring stretch

- Your hamstrings are a popular target for stretches.

- Sit on the ground with your legs extended in front of you to complete. Reaching forward with your hands toward your toes while bending forward from the belly or chest until the backs of your legs feel stretched.
- 30 seconds of holding, followed by 30 seconds of resting while re-seated. Finish it twice more.

4. Exercise all your strength.

You ought to exert more physical effort while exercising to improve. You want to push yourself over your comfort zone when you push yourself, but you don't want to push yourself too far and risk injuries like strain, sprain, or tears.

With more range of motion and flexibility as a result, this enables your body to establish a new normal.

Example:

Squatting: Pushing your thighs flat and below parallel while using a lightweight or none at all will develop the strength and range of motion of your muscles. Your range of motion will expand and build as a result of incorporating this change for 1 set after each completed exercise.

5. Bodywork and deep tissue massage
Your muscles may become restricted or tight as a result of tension buildup; massage therapy can help to relieve these symptoms. Your muscles will move more freely as a result, increasing their range of motion as well as their flexibility.

One of the best ways to promote muscle movement and de-stress the muscle, which will help you increase your range of motion, is to visit a qualified massage therapist who can isolate the specific portions of the muscles that are producing the most tension.

By boosting blood flow to muscles, reducing knots (which are thought to be inflammation or microtrauma to muscle fibers that can restrict ROM), and making fascia more malleable, massage can help muscles relax. Connective tissue called fascia creates a web-like covering for everybody's compartment.

6. Motion

In addition to having a significant impact on your joints and muscles, movement is crucial for daily function and well-being. Our muscles and joints move more when we move, which helps to improve mobility and prevents the loss of range of motion.

A daily walk of 15 to 30 minutes at a brisk pace helps to relax your muscles, improve blood flow (which aids in healing), and begin to build up your body's strength and range of motion.

Incorporating a 15–30 minute brisk walk each day can help reduce the amount of time we spend sitting and have a significant positive influence on our overall health and wellness, which includes our range of motion.

7. Increase water consumption

Water consumption is crucial for maintaining good health, as we all know. However, it's also thought that downing enough water will help to boost your ROM.

Water is present and necessary in tendons, ligaments, and muscles, so maintaining sufficient hydration can enhance muscular performance. The lubrication provided by water can make tissues and joints more pliable.

Chapter 2

Integrating More Activity to Your Daily Life Naturally

Humans' sedentary lifestyles have evolved from their migratory origins. People are accustomed to sitting in today's society. We commute to work in the automobile, spend the day seated at a desk, drive home, and then sit on the couch to watch television. And practically every day we repeat this action. On weekends, perhaps, we switch things up, get more active, and run errands.

It's not enough to make this small movement.

This sedentary way of life has been connected to several health problems, including heart disease, obesity, diabetes, and depression. Muscle deterioration, weight gain, and back and neck pain are further side effects of extended sitting. The doctor of the future won't prescribe medication; instead, he or she will educate the patient on the benefits of healthy eating, exercise, and access to fresh air.

It's always good to work out, but recent research has revealed that even a rigorous exercise program cannot undo the harm caused by prolonged sitting. Although working exercise is a fantastic idea, it's equally crucial to move around during the day.

Start moving now, whatever you do.

It's good for both your physical and emotional wellness to move your body each day. Movement enhances your overall well-being by enhancing your blood circulation, digestion, flexibility, joint health, weight management, sleep quality, productivity, and creativity. It also lowers stress levels, increases mental clarity, improves focus and concentration, and makes you feel better overall.

Throughout the Day, Here Are 17 Ways to Move:

1. Walk around. Take a podcast with you while you walk your dog or a friend or anything that inspires you.
2. Practice stretching or yoga. Moving the body in this way is soothing. Go slowly, spread a mat, and make a move. If you're stiff or uncomfortable from sitting, it's also a terrific method to move.
3. A store's entrance should be far from where you park your car. Try parking a bit more distance from the spot than normal whether you are going to work or running errands. With greater movement throughout the day, you'll be able to take more steps.
4. Have a lot of water. You will need to use the restroom more frequently if you drink more water, which will encourage you to get up and move around.
5. Make an alarm to get up, move about, and stretch once each hour. Sometimes we can become so absorbed in what we are doing that we forget to take a break and wind up sitting for a long time.

6. Playtime can be had with children or a dog. Walk or run around with your kids outside while you play fetch.

7. Dance around your home while your favorite song is playing. Unwind and enjoy yourself. When no one is looking, dance!

8. A good time to get moving is during shows or commercial breaks. Move slowly while doing sit-ups and stretches.

9. When feasible, use the stairs. The difficulty may increase if you work on the fifteenth level of a building. However, if you're fatigued, take the elevator after a few flights of stairs and then continue walking. Walking the stairs is preferable if you need to ascend a few flights.

10. During your lunch break, take a brief stroll. Take a ten-minute stroll around your workplace complex after you eat. Sitting down again for the afternoon will assist with digestion and movement.

11. While standing in line or using the restroom, perform calf lifts. You'll be surprised how frequently you'll have time

to perform calf raises while standing in line.

12. Face challenges in your own home. Short training breaks can be done anywhere, even in the gym. The counter is available for modified push-ups or planks; the stairs can be used for step-ups and balance exercises; and canned foods can be used as hand weights. It is possible to be imaginative and fun with a short challenge.

13. Cleaning. It's amazing how much cleaning can make you sweat; washing the tub may quickly become exhilarating. Take on tough stains or residue, get rid of dust bunnies, spruce up furniture, or even forego the washing machine and hand wash a few things.

14. Hold meetings while walking. When compared to sitting, some people discover that walking helps them think more clearly. Hold your walking meetings outside if at all possible.

15. Either while standing or while moving, calls are an excellent excuse to multitask

whether they are inside or outside. A target number of phone calls you'll make every day or each week could be established by you.

16. Cut down on couch time. Since couches are made to be comfortable, you will probably settle in for a while once you locate a spot that feels good. There will be a lot of movement if you sit on the floor. You'll frequently find yourself reaching for an exercise band, a physioball, a lacrosse ball, or the foam roller if you keep moving in this manner.

    Furthermore, avoid lying on an outdated or unsupportive couch. Keeping your ear, shoulder, and hip in a straight line will help you maintain good back health. Your body is frequently misaligned in all three directions when you lie on a ccouch.

17. Invest in a foam roller, tennis ball, or lacrosse ball. Many various parts of your body, particularly the legs and back, can be relieved of stress using these tools. Depending on the intensity you want and

the body parts you want to target, there are a variety of foam roller shapes and sizes to pick from.

Your everyday regimen must include mobility. You may easily begin and maintain these attainable and sustainable measures.

Even though establishing that pattern may be challenging, once you do, you will feel much better. To balance out your sedentary lifestyle, use creativity and some movement.

Chapter 3

Managing Sedentary Behaviors

Even if contemporary advancements make life easier, many of us now lead more sedentary lifestyles. The obesity pandemic is thought to be mostly attributed to people sitting down more often and moving less. This is linked to several health issues. It takes some intentional effort to change a sedentary lifestyle at first, but the rewards of increasing physical activity are numerous and well worth the effort.

Here are some suggestions to help you begin moving, whether you work at a desk all day or are just finding it difficult to get motivated.

Walking more
The health advantages of a daily 30-minute walk have been amply demonstrated by the study. Even at the office, it's simple to start moving around more. Instead of sitting at a conference table, suggest having meetings outside. A longer dog

walk is one more action you could attempt before or after work.

Seek additional occasions to go for a stroll. As an illustration, if you live close enough, consider having your children walk to or from school, or at the very least, to the bus stop. Making it a family activity, you might even go for a walk after supper.

Use the Stairs

Jogging burns fewer calories per minute than stair climbing, which is regarded as vigorous-intensity exercise.

You may develop and maintain strong bones, joints, and muscles by using the stairs whenever you can. This will also help you to keep a healthy weight.

Spatter the Parking Lot

If you can do it safely, parking your car further away from your destination in the parking lot or on the street is a simple approach to extend your day's total number of steps.

If you have the time and the physical capacity to go a little further, you will reap the benefits of more exercise, just like when you choose to use the stairs rather than the elevator.

It also provides you a chance to spend some time outside enjoying the sunshine or the changing of the seasons, which can be beneficial for your mental health. You can stroll across the parking lot or around the block from your office.

Quit Driving
In the present era, the amount of overweight and obesity is correlated with how we travel. Active modes of transportation, like cycling or walking, provide significant health advantages over more passive modes and have a stronger ability to prevent obesity.

Even using public transportation instead of driving to work seems to be connected with a lower body mass index (BMI). Compared to simply strolling from your front door to your garage, standing on a metro platform, or traveling to a bus stop involves more steps. But even if you do drive your car, you might be able to fit in those extra steps if you live in a city where you have to park in a lot or a few blocks from your home.

During Work

Your workday may not need to include more activity if it is physically taxing. But adding more activity can be a significant way of life change for those who spend their days sitting at a computer.

Rise

If your job necessitates prolonged sitting, make it a point to stand up at least once every 20 minutes. Particularly if you're prone to become engrossed in a project and losing track of time, you might need to set a reminder using your phone or calendar.

You don't necessarily have to finish what you're doing to take a quick standing or stretching break, so don't be concerned if you're worried about stopping your workflow. It's simple to peruse printed documents while standing up or answering calls.

Instead of writing an email, consider taking short breaks away from your desk to drink some water or speak with a coworker at their workstation.

Switch Up Your Workstation
Additionally, you can think about acquiring a standing desk, a treadmill workstation, or a fitness ball seat (which encourages "active sitting," in which you use your core). Even some of your everyday computer work can be done while standing up if your workstation can be changed to different heights.

Examine a fitness tracker
With the use of a pedometer, you can easily keep track of your daily activity by monitoring your steps.

Realizing how active you are will help you see trends or behaviors that point toward a life that is too sedentary. Finding opportunities to move more will help you combat the negative consequences of prolonged sitting.

You can measure calories in and out, your daily activity level, and your objectives with sophisticated fitness trackers. They do more than just count your steps. Even your heart rate and sleep are monitored by some.

Many smartphone apps offer similar features, so you don't even need a wearable fitness tracker if that's not your style or your budget. You won't need to remember to log your activities because numerous solutions are free and may passively track them.

Construct engaging pastimes
Your life can be made more active by finding fun activities that keep you active.

In the house

After a hard day at work, resist the urge to crash by continuing to move and attempting to persuade yourself to stay active until you get home.

Making time for exercise after supper not only improves your fitness but also lowers your risk of developing insulin resistance, helps keep blood sugar levels in the ideal range, and keeps your metabolism running smoothly.

Chapter 4

Fussy Eaters': No-Fuss Nutrition Guide

It's a bit more difficult than teaching our tiny ones their ABCs to get them to comprehend the details of a nutritious diet. However, a good place to start is with the foundations! To support their developing bodies, children need a diet that is well-balanced and nutrient-rich. This will also give them a head start on feeling good and maximizing their enjoyment of food and life.

Use this easy nutrition guide to explain to your kids the benefits of eating nutritious food for the entire family.

In terms of nutrition, there are six major categories:

1. Water, lipids (fats and oils), proteins, and carbohydrates make up the macronutrients.

2. Minerals and vitamins comprise the Micronutrients.

Compared to adults, children have different nutritional needs, so in a perfect world, your child would consume (every day):

Vegetables with color
- 4-5 servings of root veggies, whole grains, and dairy products
- Eggs, fish, poultry, beef, and beans: 2 50% serves
- 1 serving of fruit
- 1-2 servings of dairy, if tolerated
- Wild on Veggies, Mild on Fruit

A child's diet must include vegetables rich in minerals, vitamins, and fiber. But there is frequent opposition to this important dietary group. Get your toddler used to eating vegetables every day by setting up a schedule for them. Vegetables can be cleverly masked by including them in baked goods. Healthy muffins or cakes can be made by blending vegetables like beetroot, carrot, and zucchini.

Fruit is also essential for your youngster because it contains necessary vitamins and minerals and is a far healthier option than candy. Although fruit can have high sugar content, it should still be consumed in moderation and different ways.

The best method to help your child develop a positive relationship with food is by teaching them about the origins of the food we eat. Everyone will benefit from the fresh product by helping to build a vegetable garden or even a herb garden, which is a terrific way to involve the whole family.

Go Whole Grain If You're Using Grains!
To give young children the energy they need to function throughout the day, carbohydrates are recommended. When compared to their processed and refined cousins, such as white bread, which has had its nutrient-rich outer layers scraped away during processing, whole grains

and root vegetables offer higher levels of fiber, vitamins, minerals, and antioxidants. The Glycemic Index of these whole food options is lower, which means that your child will digest and absorb their food's energy much more gradually. High GI foods cause blood sugar levels to surge and can cause erratic moods.

It can be difficult to encourage your toddler to recognize the beauty of meals with earthy tones. It's critical to add appealing low-sugar items, like minimally processed peanut butter, to your child's lunch box because while packing it with carrot sticks or wholegrain bread is a wonderful start, it might not go over well.

Fats are Beneficial
The idea that everything containing fat is negative is a common misconception concerning fats. For a balanced diet, healthy fats are not only possible but also necessary. Docosahexaenoic acid (DHA), an omega-3 essential fatty acid that is necessary for good health but that the body is unable to produce, is present in a few certain

types of lipids. To receive DHA, one needs to consume food sources or take supplements. Incorporating a children's flavor-flavored DHA supplement into their diet may be the best option because getting your child to eat fish, a strong source of DHA may cause some conflict.

Calcium-rich dairy products
To aid in the development of children's strong, healthy bones and teeth, calcium is regarded as a crucial component of a balanced diet. Most kids would benefit from consuming one to four glasses of milk each day, depending on their age, especially if they are not consuming any other high-calcium foods. Even better, if your youngster doesn't enjoy eating meat, the majority of dairy products are a great source of protein and a great supply of calcium.

Incorporate milk alternatives, like almonds, seeds, and even greens if you can find a pleasant way to serve them, into their diet if it becomes an issue. It's a good idea to offer smoothies that are packed with fruit and their preferred yogurt, and soy products with calcium addition occasionally work.

Components of proteins

To assemble wholesome muscle and tissue, the body requires protein. Lean meats, eggs, poultry, legumes, fish, nuts, and cheese are all sources of protein. At least twice a week, pick low-fat cuts of meat, poultry, or shellfish. When looking for ways to boost their protein intake, beans, and peas are also fantastic choices. Additionally, you have the choice of adding nuts to your favorite yogurt, cereal, or veggie dish or you can try purchasing a nut butter spread.

In the past, 'extras' like chips, lollipops, cookies, chocolate, etc. were frequently permitted within the rules published by various bodies that issue dietary advice. However, they are beginning to disappear as the drive to promote healthy eating and highlight "real" foods with nutritional value catches up with the difficult work at hand for mothers everywhere: Giving their children the very best start and habits to live by in life.

Chapter 5

Basic Breathing Techniques for Reducing Tension and Pain

It only takes a few minutes and is portable to use this stress-relieving breathing method. If it becomes a regular part of your daily routine, you will reap the greatest rewards. You can carry it out while standing, sitting in a back-supporting chair, reclining on a bed, or lying on a yoga mat on the floor.

Do your best to put yourself at ease. Any clothing that is preventing you from breathing easily should be taken off. Laying down, position your arms with your palms up and slightly out from your sides. Your feet should be flat on the ground while your legs should be straight or slightly bent. Your arms should be on the chair arms if you are seated.

Put both of your feet flat on the ground whether you're standing or sitting. Put your feet about hip-width apart, wherever you are standing.

- Without trying to force it, allow your breath to go as deep into your belly as is comfortable.
- Try taking a few breaths through your nose and then exhaling through your mouth.
- Take frequent, gentle breaths in. A steady count from 1 to 5 can be beneficial for certain people. Initially, you could have trouble getting to 5.
- If you find this helpful, gently release it after counting from 1 to 5 once more.
- For at least 5 minutes, continue doing this.

Pain-relieving Breathing Exercises

Learning how to relax using breathing techniques is one of the best things patients can do to help lower the stress in their lives.

Because deep breathing signals the brain to relax and quiet down, deep breathing helps reduce stress in the body. This message is then communicated to the body by the brain. Additionally, deep breathing lowers some of the physiological effects of stress, including elevated blood pressure, a faster heartbeat, and rapid breathing.

Exercises for breathing are also simple to learn, which is another benefit. No additional equipment or tools are required, and patients are free to perform them whenever they wish. Patients might also experiment with various workouts to find which ones are most effective.

There are alternative approaches, such as integrating breathing with activities like yoga, images, and meditation, which are not included in the methods that follow.

Belly Breath

Belly breathing is the name of the initial exercise, which is straightforward to understand and simple to perform. Starting there is the best course of action, particularly for people who have never practiced breathing exercises. All of these exercises can aid patients in unwinding and reducing tension, even though the other ones are more difficult.

Simple and incredibly calming belly breathing techniques exist. Whenever they need to unwind or reduce tension, patients can attempt this simple activity.

- Lie back in a relaxed position.
- Placing one hand on your chest and the other on the area of your belly right below your ribs will help.
- By inhaling deeply through your nose, allow your stomach to push your hand away. You should not flinch at all.
- Taking a whistling motion with your lips pursed, exhale. Push all of the air out with the hand that is inserted into your tummy.

Repeat 3–10 times this breathing exercise. With each breath, take it slowly.

Patients might choose to give one of the following more difficult breathing techniques a try once they've mastered belly breathing.

4 - 8 breaths

Both sitting and lying down can be used to perform this exercise, which also employs belly breathing.

- Beginning with the belly breathing exercise, place one hand on your abdomen and the other on your chest.
- As you inhale slowly and deeply, count aloud from 1 to 4 in your head.
- Silently count from 1 to 7 while holding your breath.
- Count silently from 1 to 8 while completely exhaling. When you count to eight, make an effort to expel all of your air.
- To feel at ease, repeat 3–7 times.

Breathing in rolls

Developing full lung capacity and concentrating on breathing rhythm are the goals of roll breathing. Any position will work, but lying on your back with your knees bent is the best for learning.

- Your right hand should be on your chest, and your left hand should be on your stomach. As you breathe in and out, watch how your hands move.
- By breathing so that your "belly" (left) hand rises with each inhalation and your "chest" (right) hand stays steady, you can practice filling your lower lungs.
- Whenever you breathe in, use your nose, and whenever you exhale, use your mouth. 8–10 times should be done.
- Add the following second stage to your breathing after you have puffed and expelled your lower lungs 8 to 10 times: Continue breathing in through your upper chest after taking a few breaths into your lower lungs as you did before. Your left hand will also a tiny bit fall when you do this, and your right hand will rise as you do it.
- Make a faint, whooshing sound as your left-hand falls first, followed by your right

hand, while you gently exhale through your mouth. Feel your body relaxing more and more as you exhale, releasing any remaining tension.

Spend 3 to 5 minutes doing this type of inhalation and exhalation. Keep in mind how your chest and belly move in a way that resembles rolling waves as they rise and fall.

Up until you can do it practically anyplace, practice roll breathing every day for a few weeks. Anytime you require one, you can use it as a quick relaxing technique.

Attention: When attempting roll breathing for the first time, some person experience lightheadedness. If this occurs, take a deep breath and slowly stand up.

Consult your doctor if you have chronic pain as a result of any illness or injury! They will collaborate with you to alleviate your suffering, improve your functionality and standard of living, and help you get back to living!